The Purpose of this Book.

Clinicians are tasked daily with the responsibility of collecting pieces of information from the history, physical, and tests of a patient; to determine what specific problems the patient might have. From this a treatment plan can be devised and progress measured.

Echocardiography provides a unique non-invasive tool to help the clinician decide exactly what type of heart problem a patient might have.

In Parts 1 and 2 of this series we introduced physicians, paramedics, and nurses, to the basics of Echocardiography. The key to finding heart disease - or any health problem - is knowing what to look for and putting the pieces of the puzzle together.

In part 3, we will look at specific examples of a variety of Cardiac problems found on echocardiograms and put the pieces of the puzzle together.

Echocardiograms - Part 3: Specific Case Examples of Cardiac Disease with Echocardiographic Findings.

By: Dr. Richard M. Fleming
Physicist – Nuclear Cardiologist

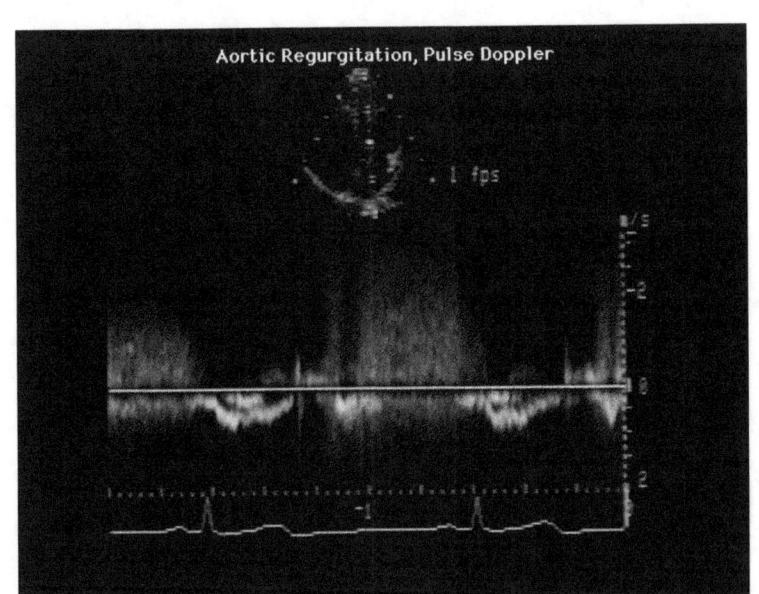
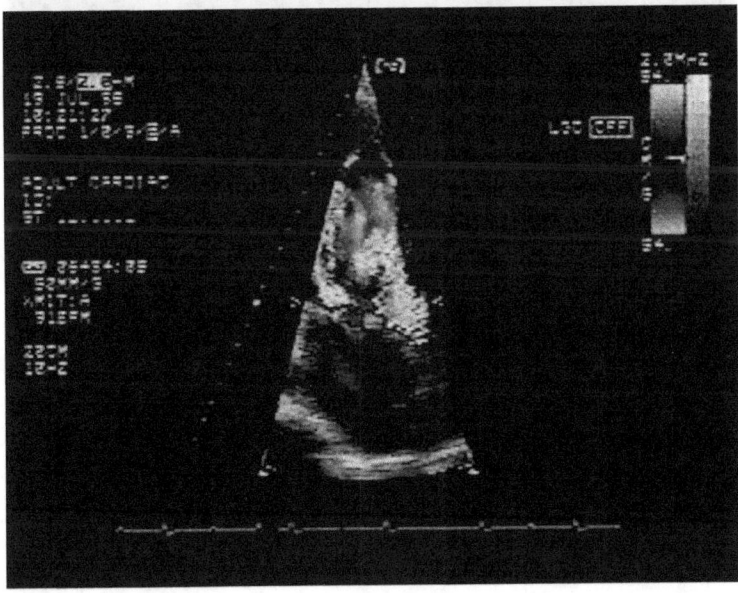

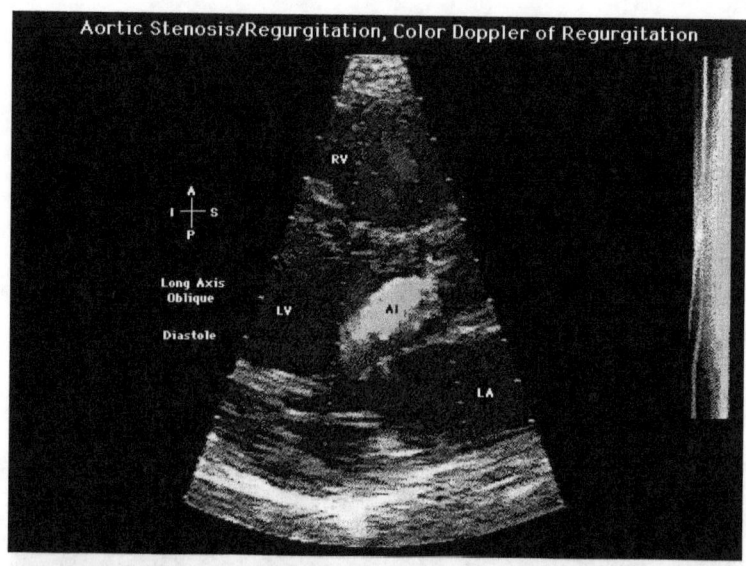

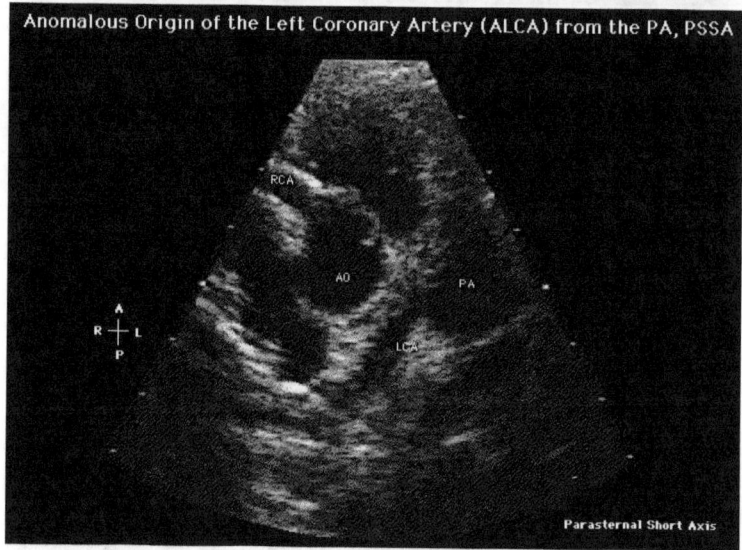

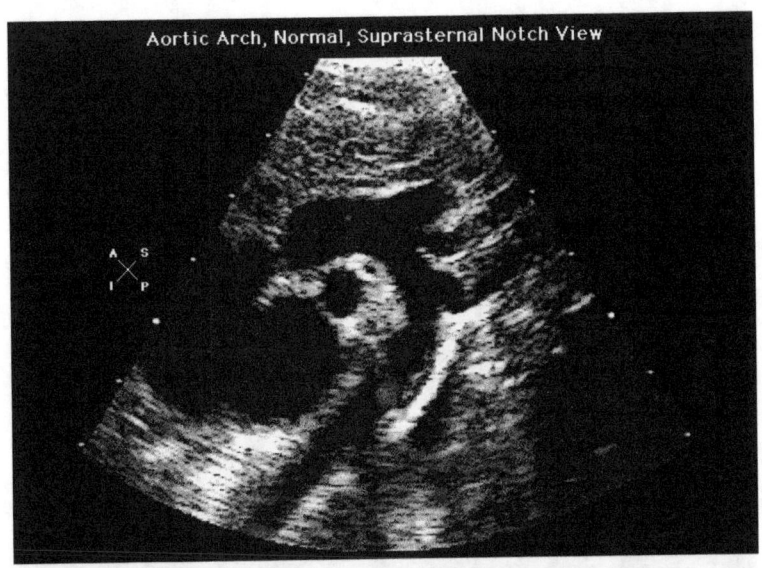

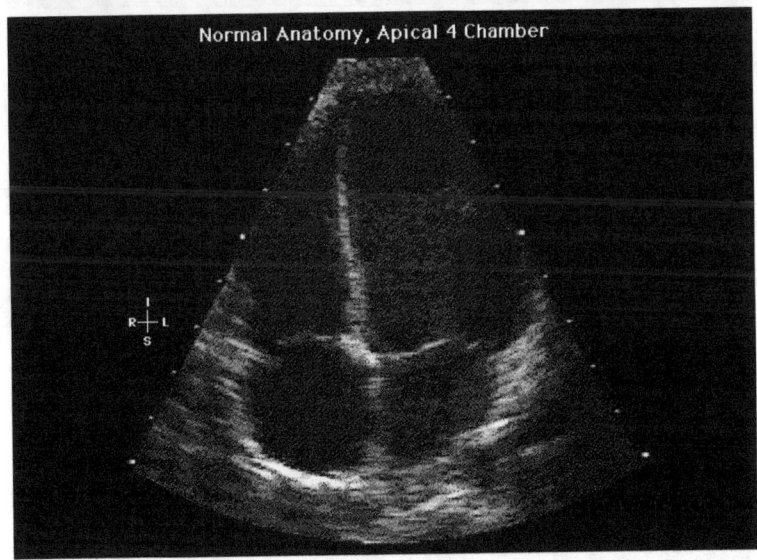

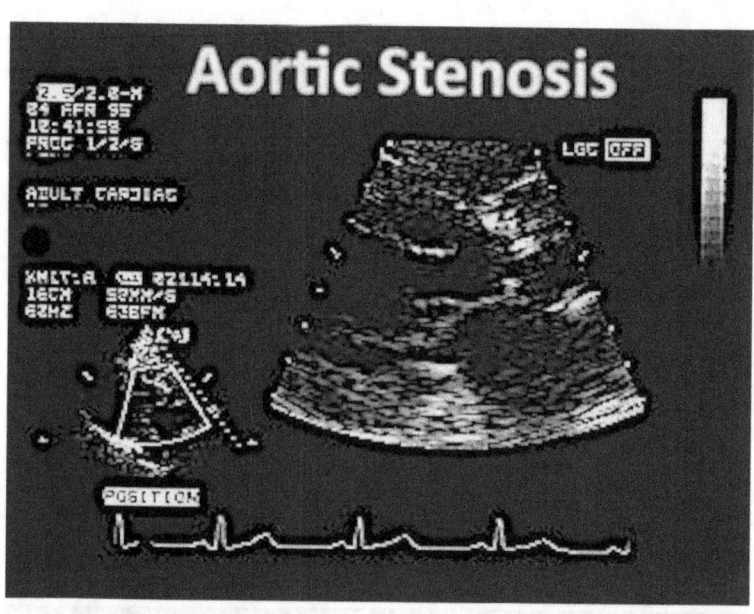

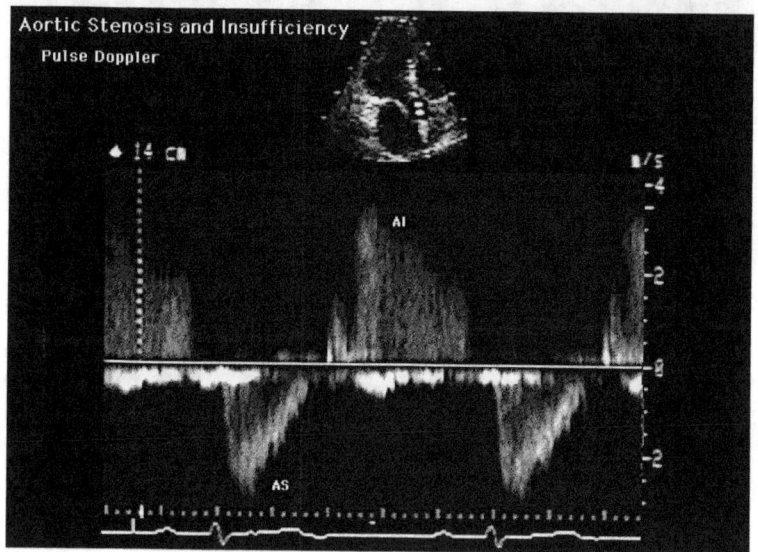

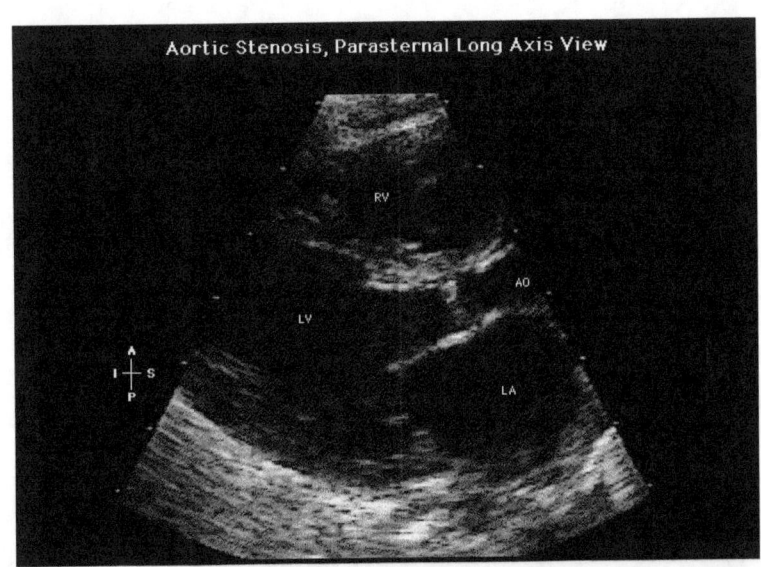

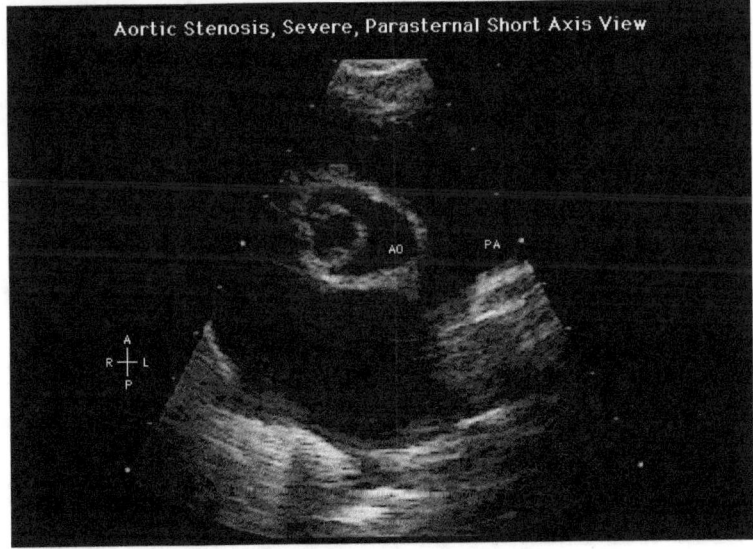

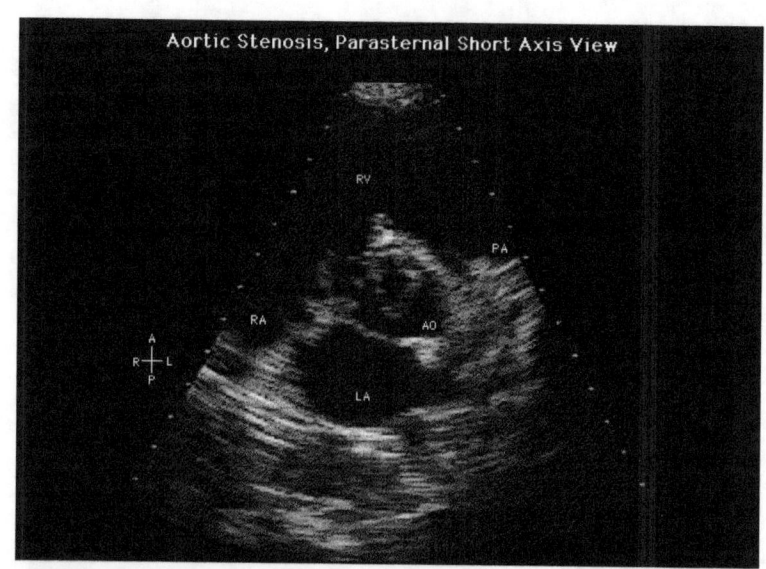

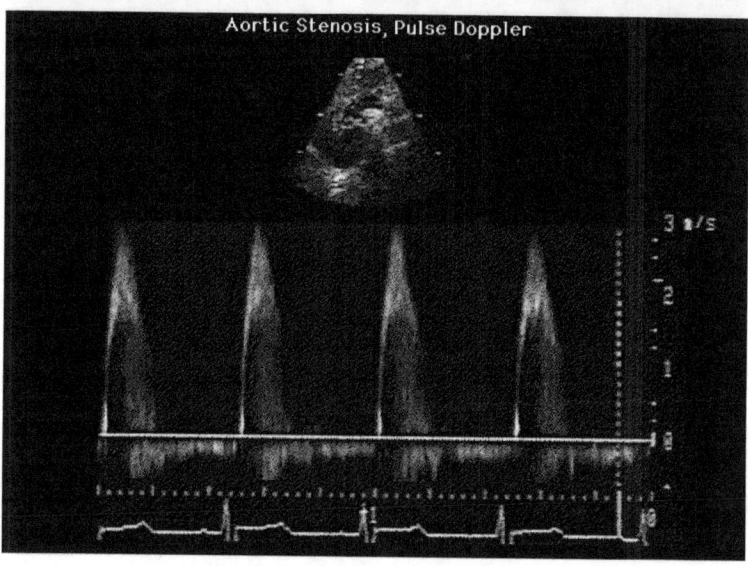

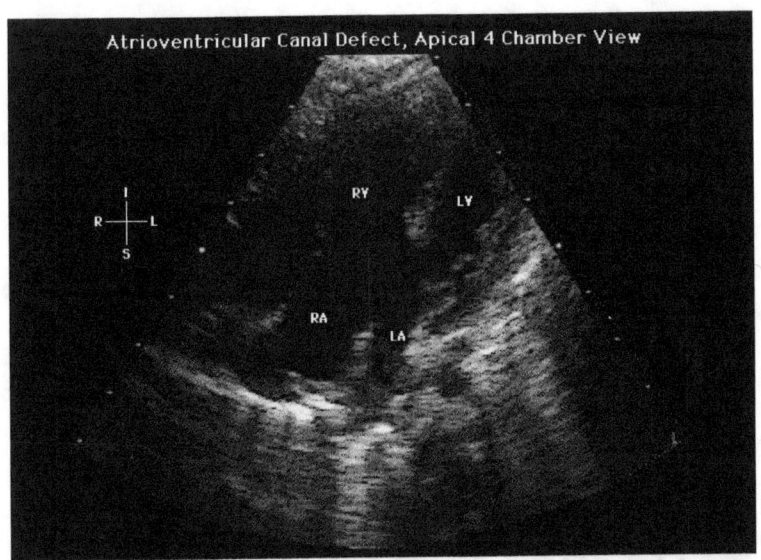

Atrioventricular Canal Defect, Apical 4 Chamber View

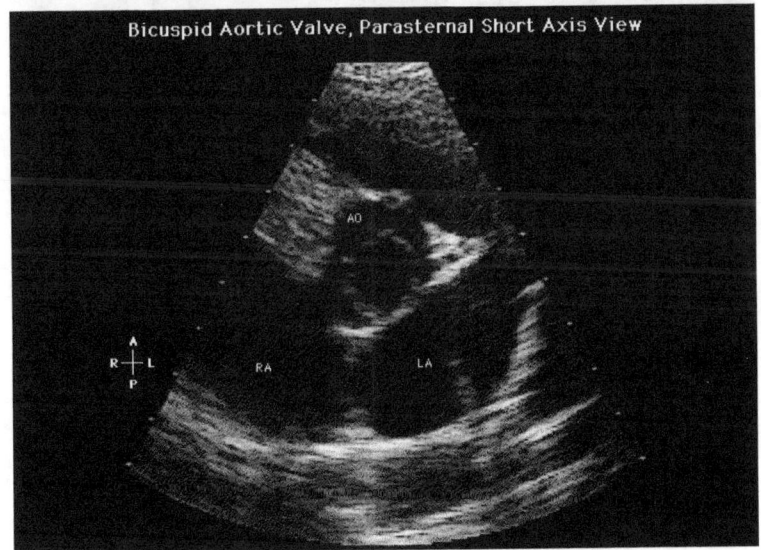

Bicuspid Aortic Valve, Parasternal Short Axis View

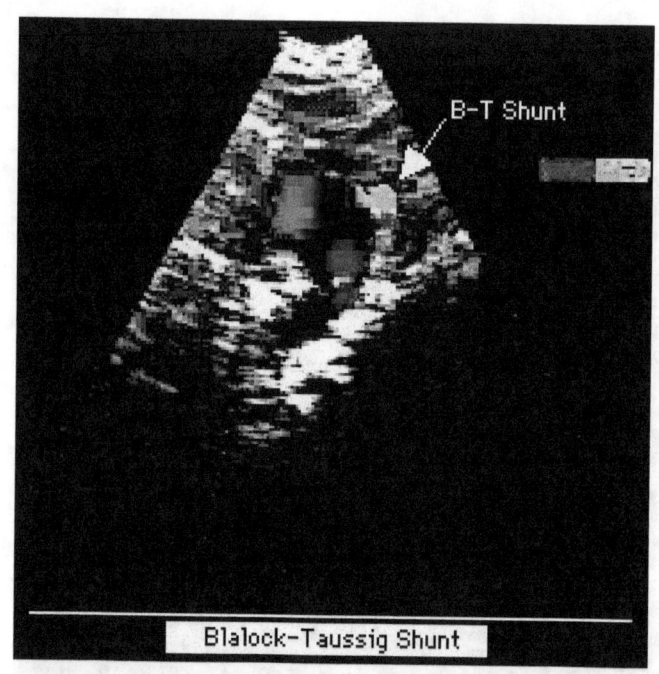

Blalock-Taussig Shunt

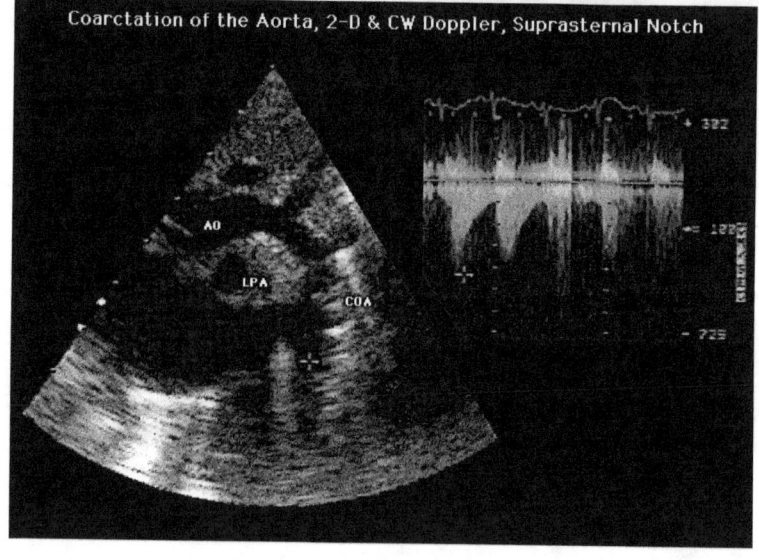

Coarctation of the Aorta, 2-D & CW Doppler, Suprasternal Notch

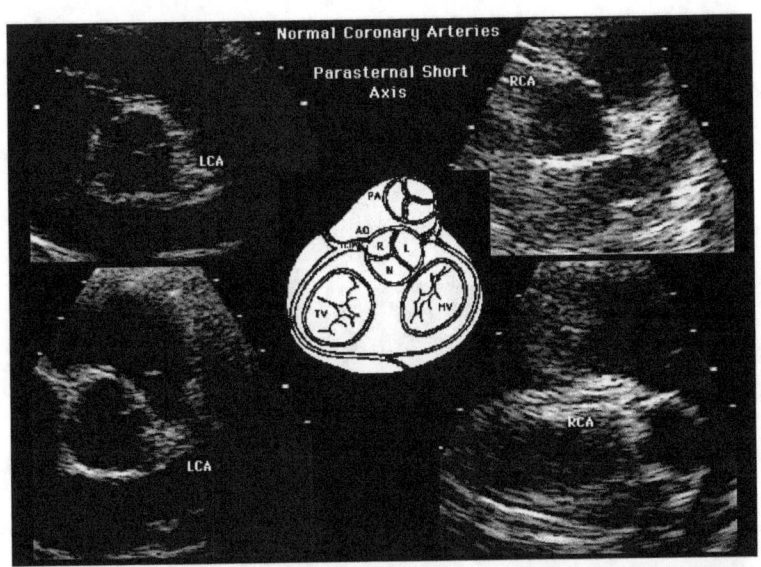

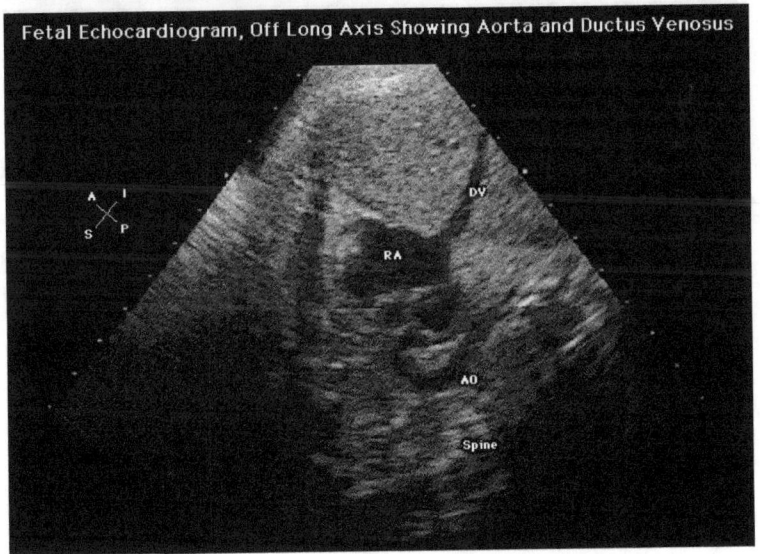

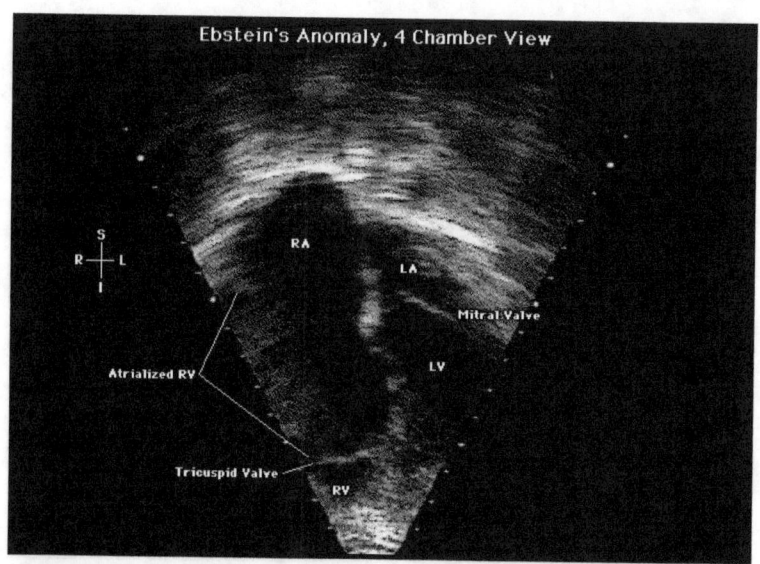

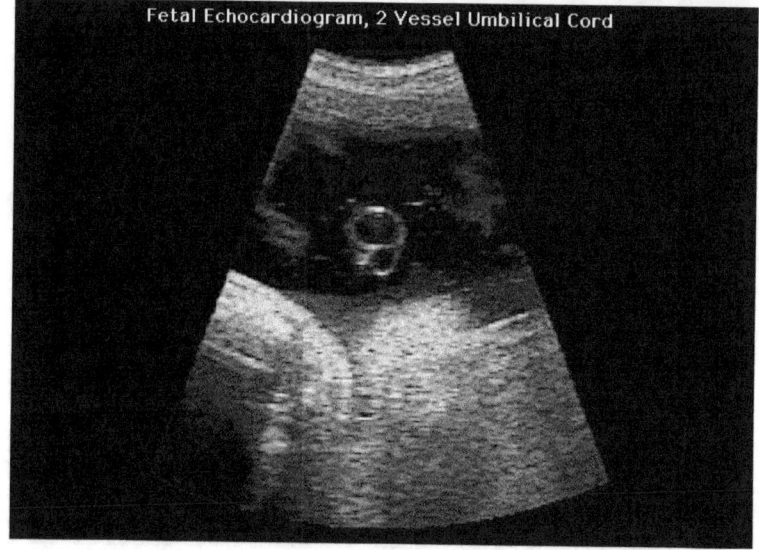

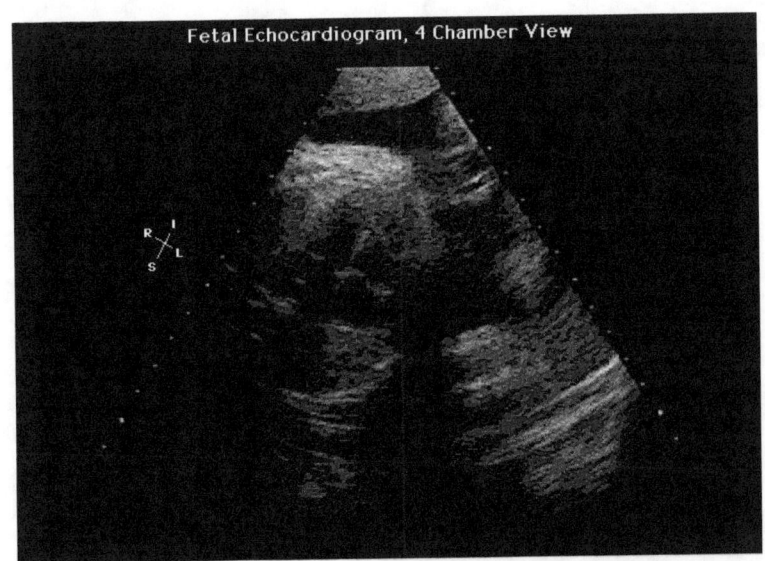

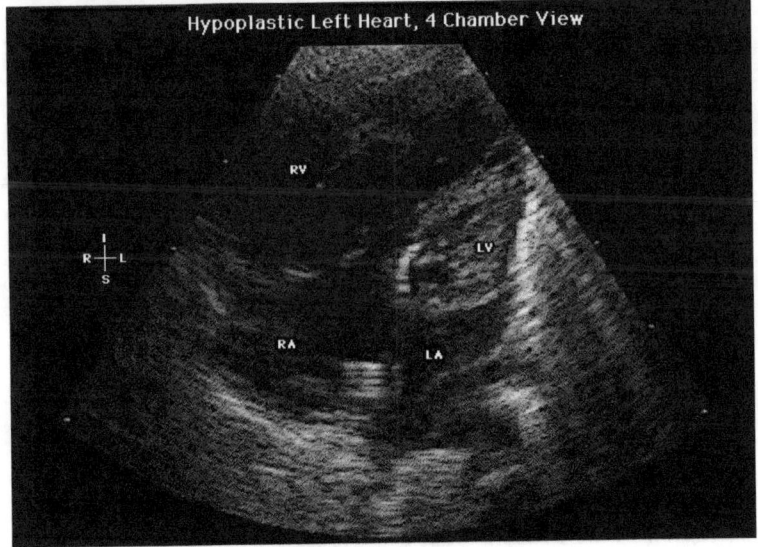

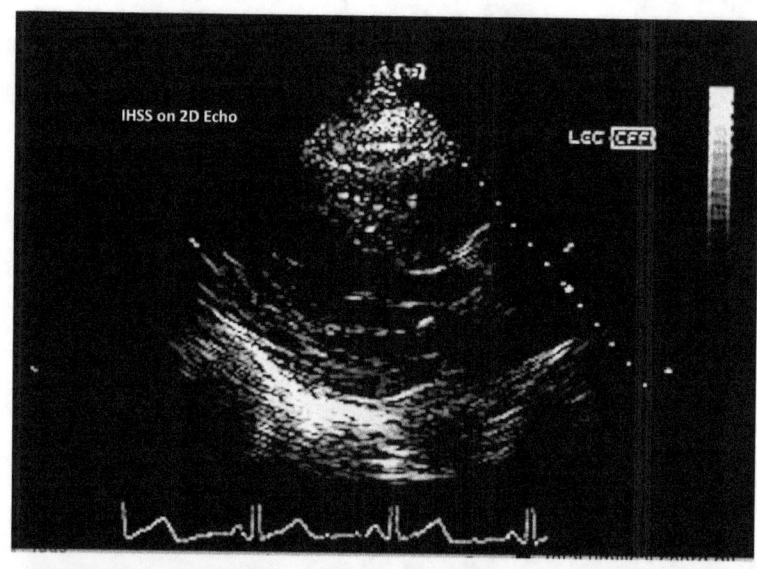
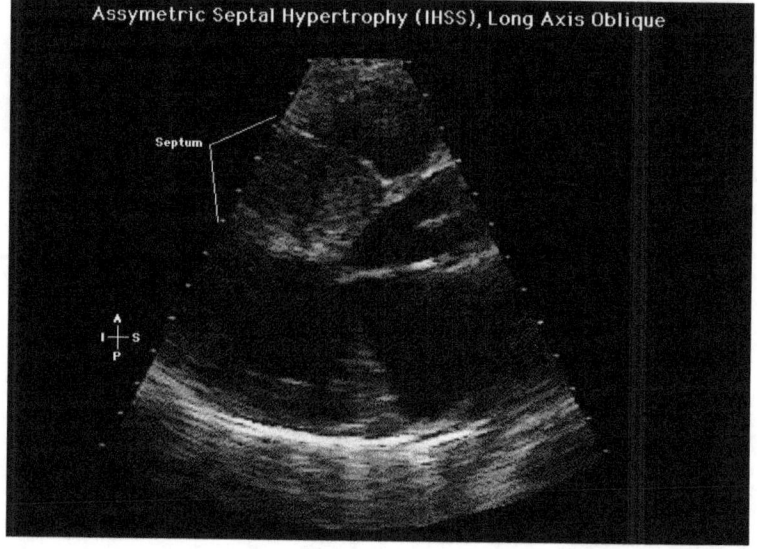

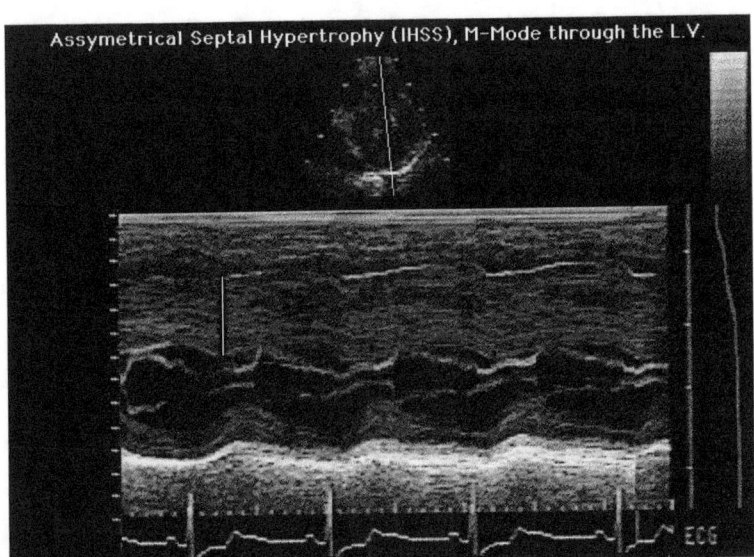

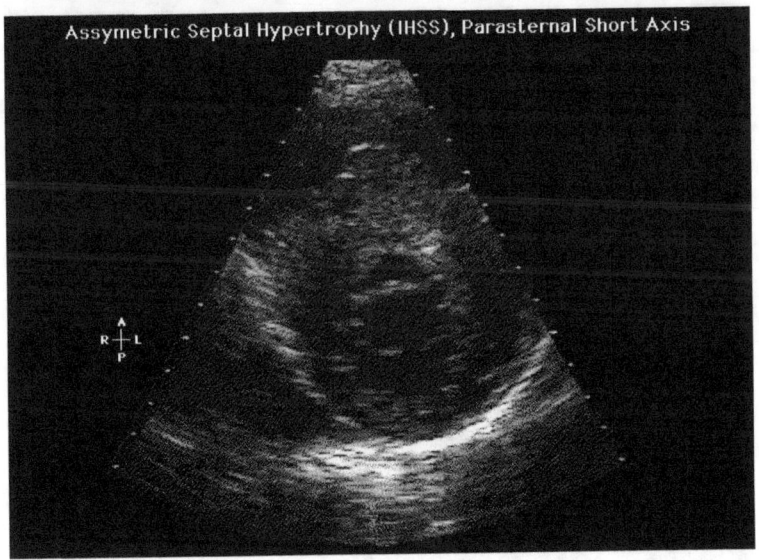

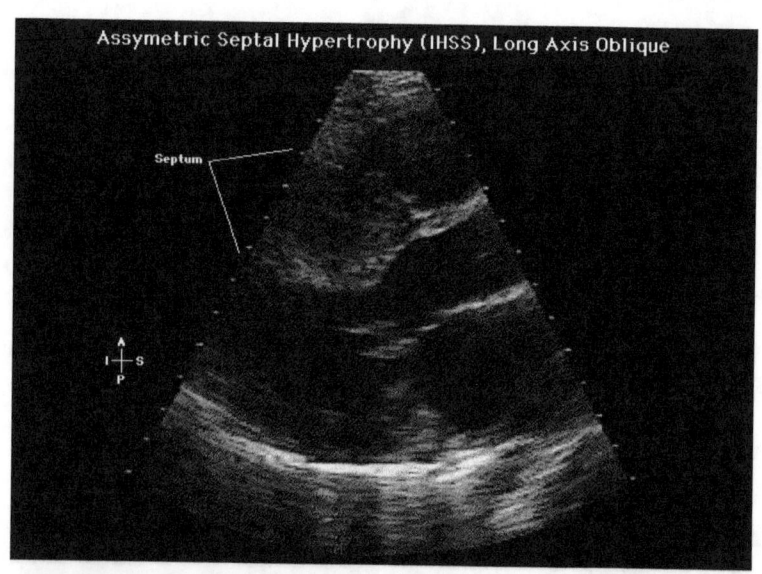
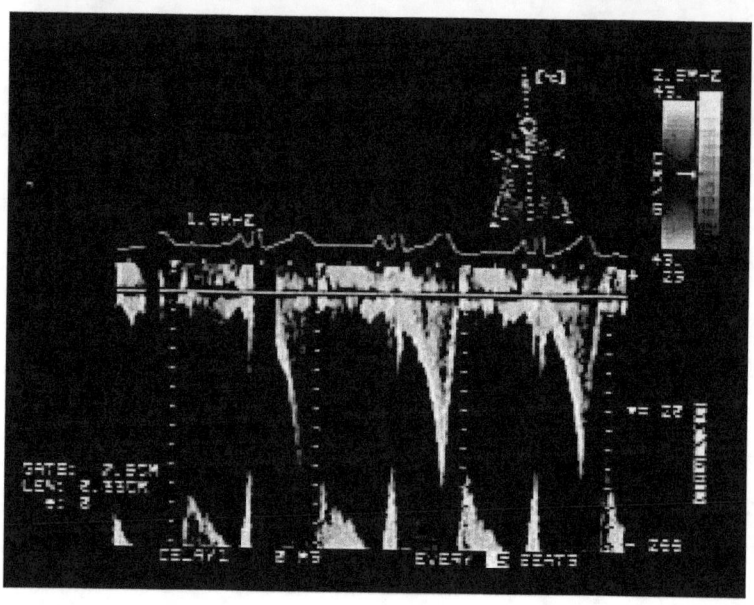

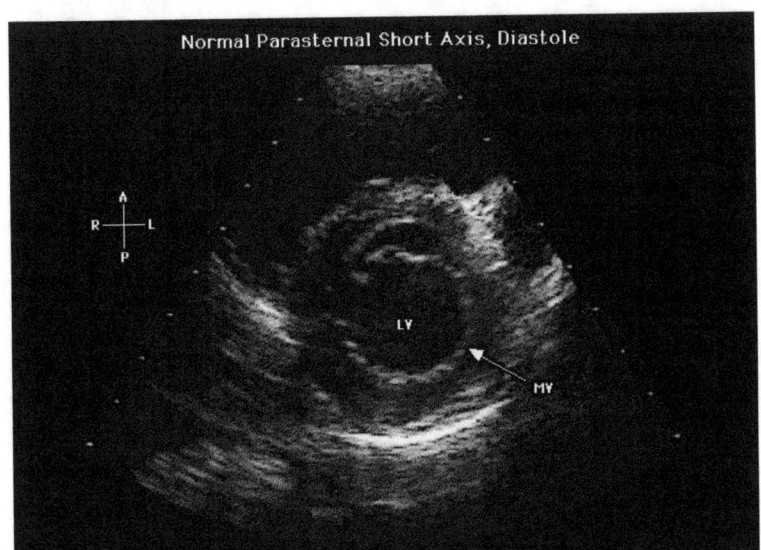
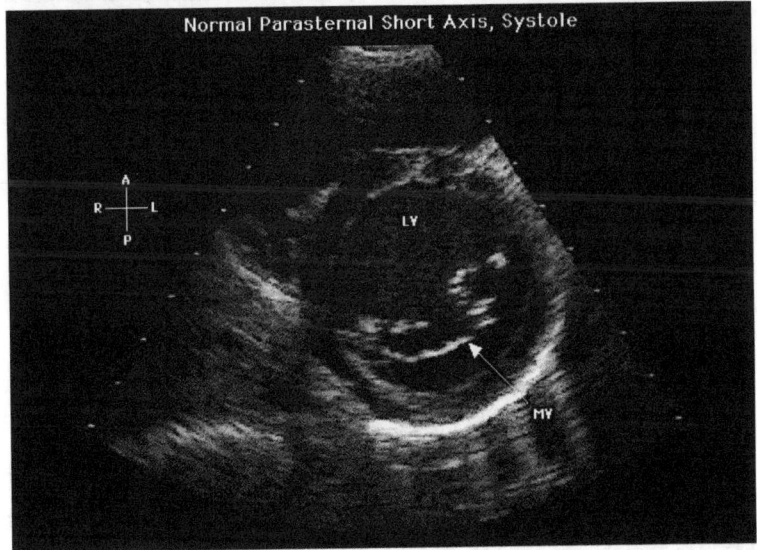

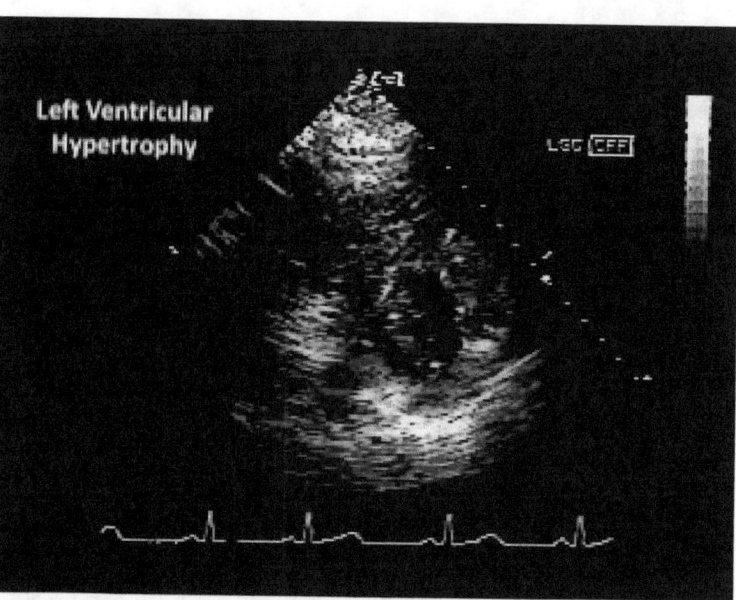

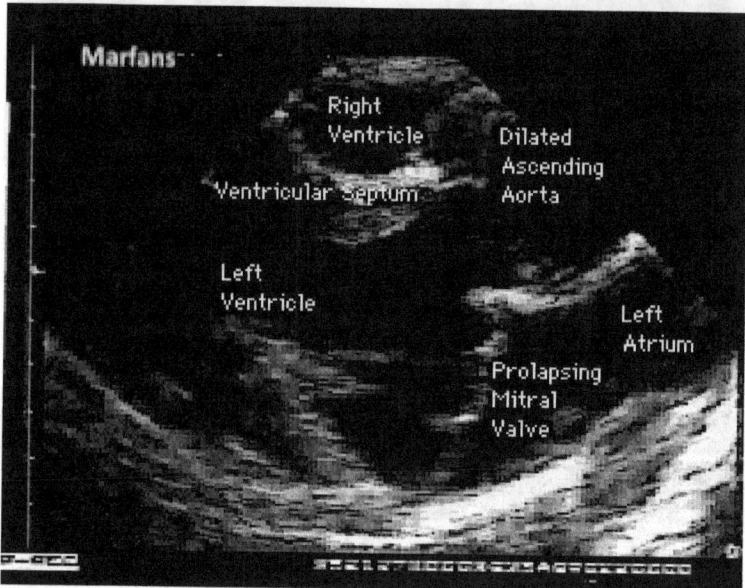

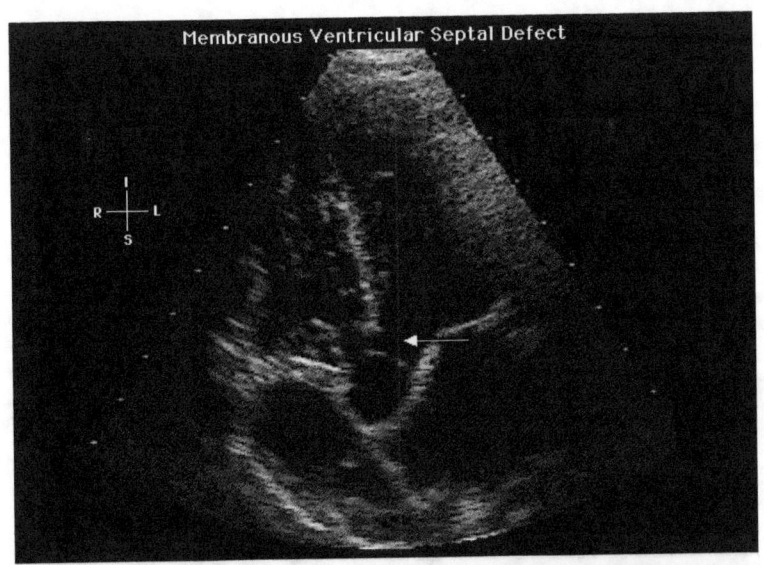

Membranous Ventricular Septal Defect

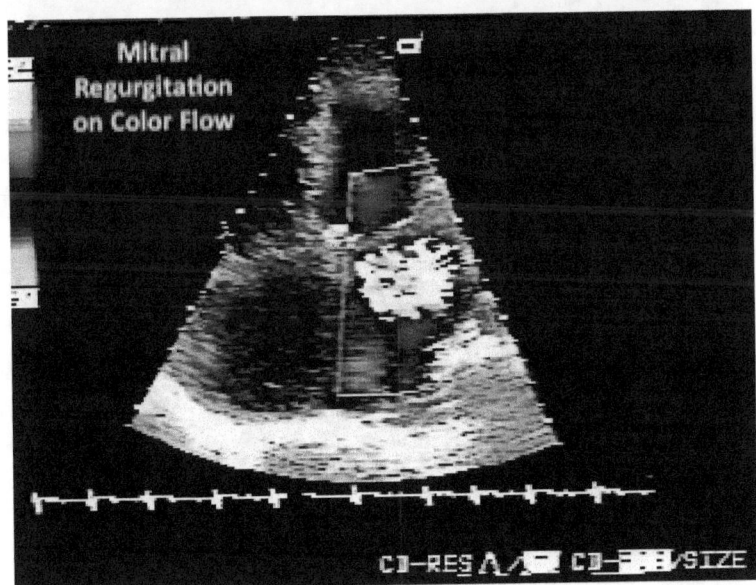

Mitral Regurgitation on Color Flow

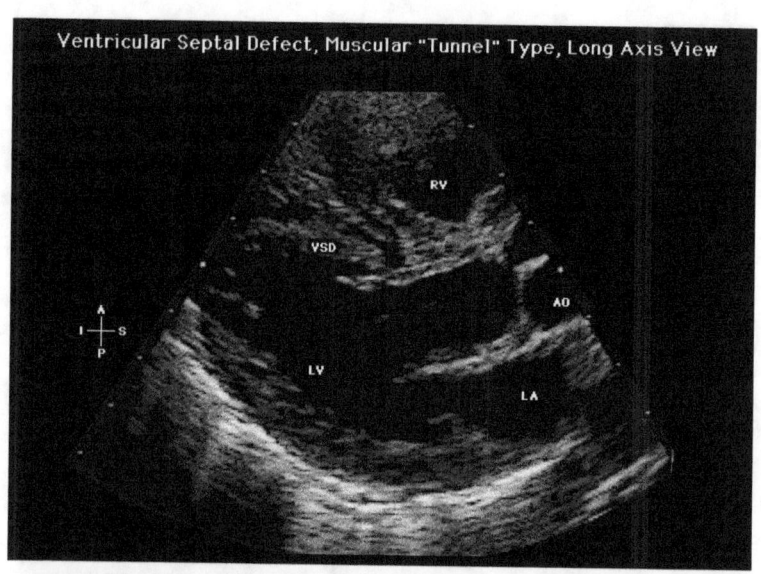

Ventricular Septal Defect, Muscular "Tunnel" Type, Long Axis View

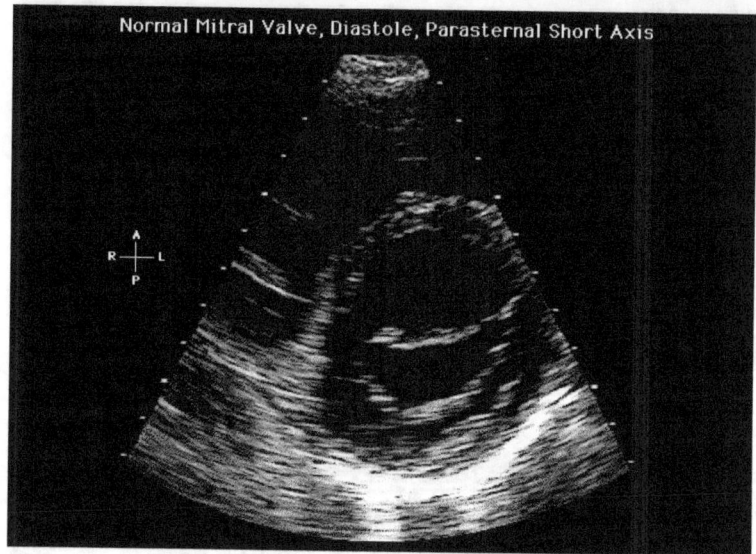

Normal Mitral Valve, Diastole, Parasternal Short Axis

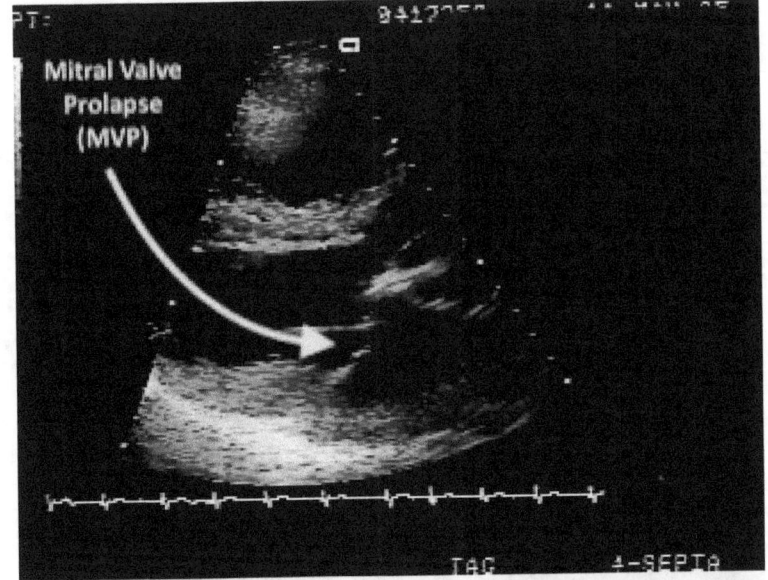

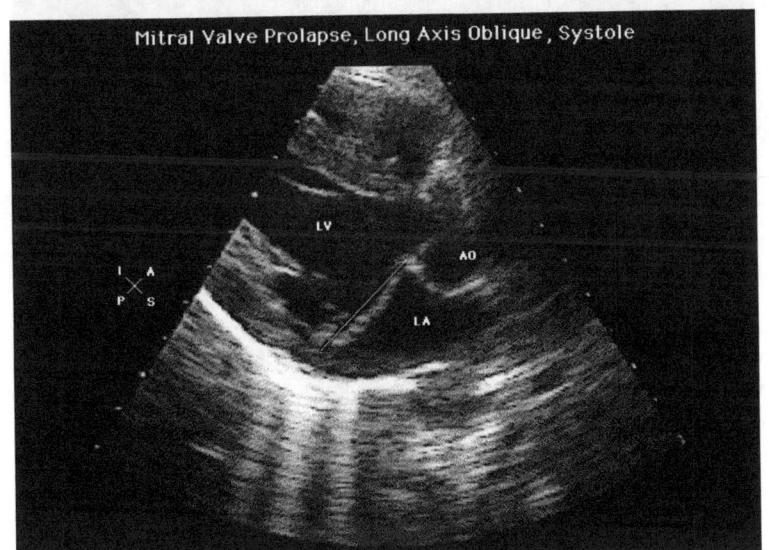

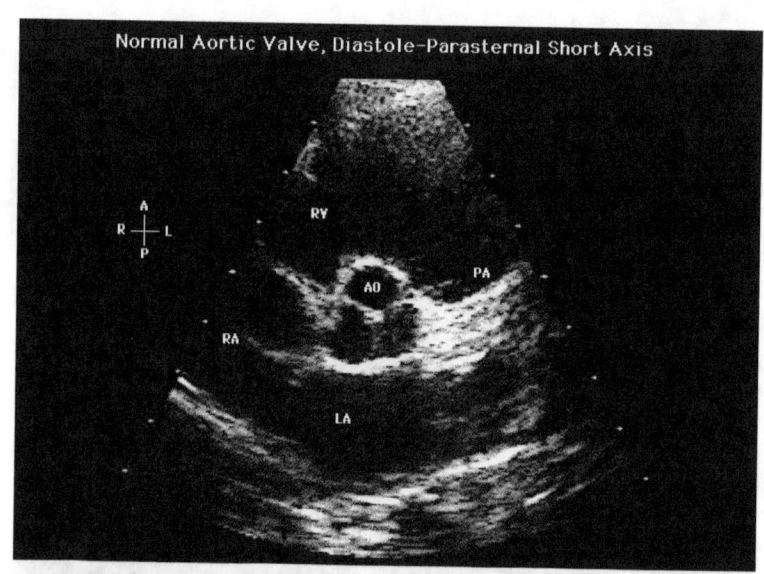

Normal Aortic Valve, Diastole–Parasternal Short Axis

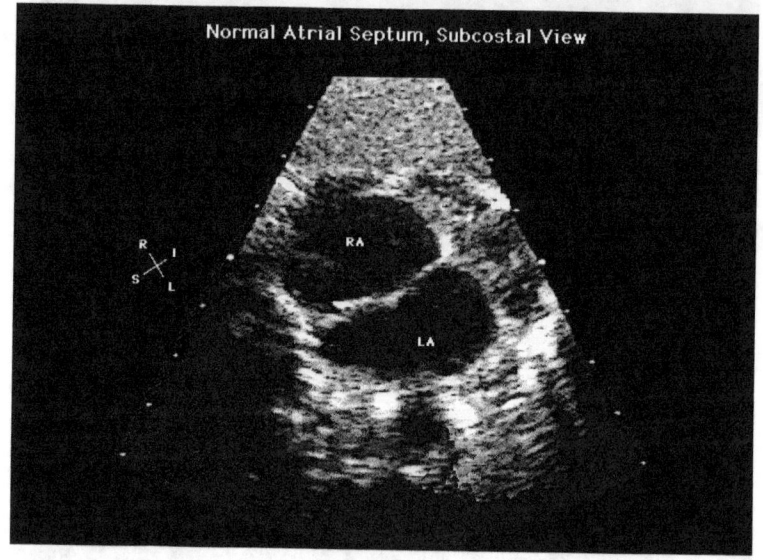

Normal Atrial Septum, Subcostal View

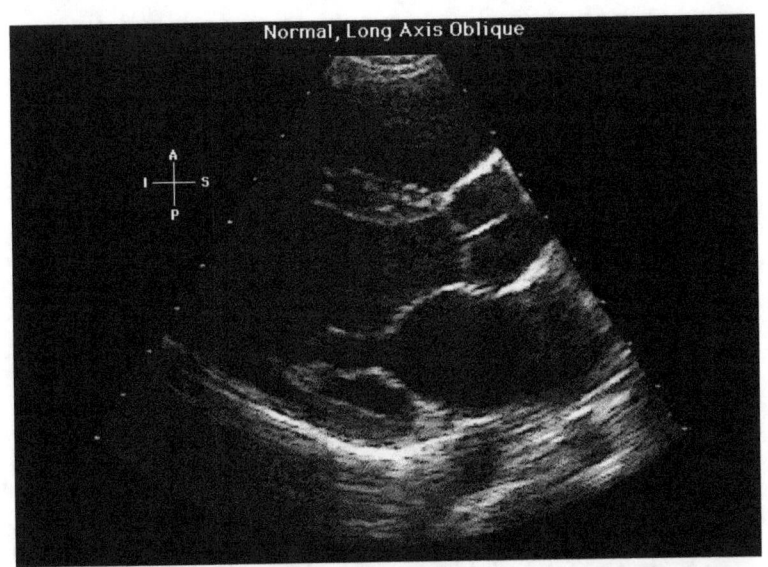

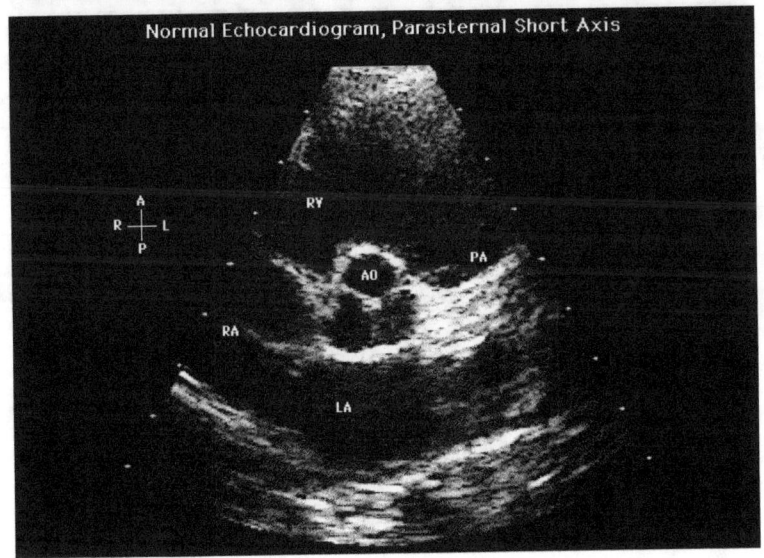

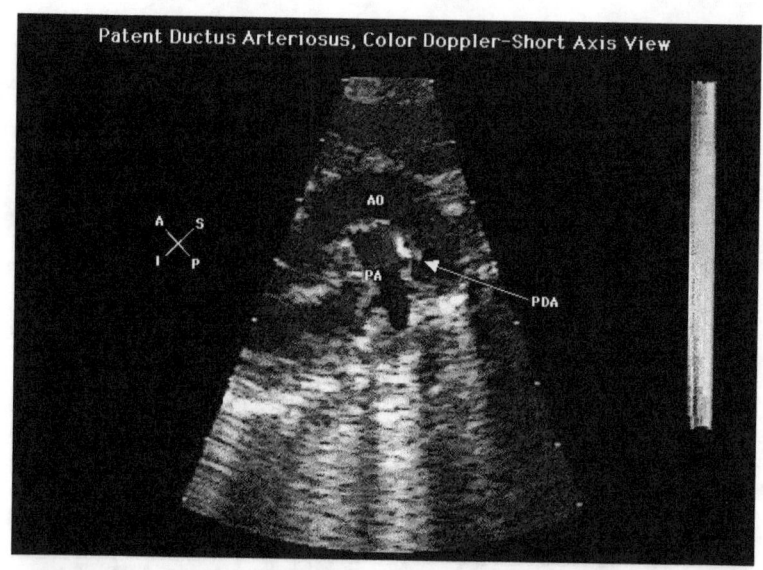

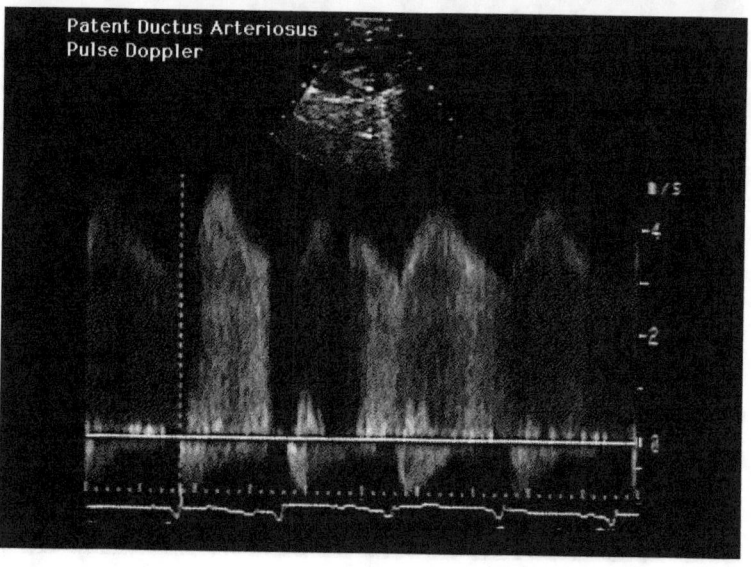

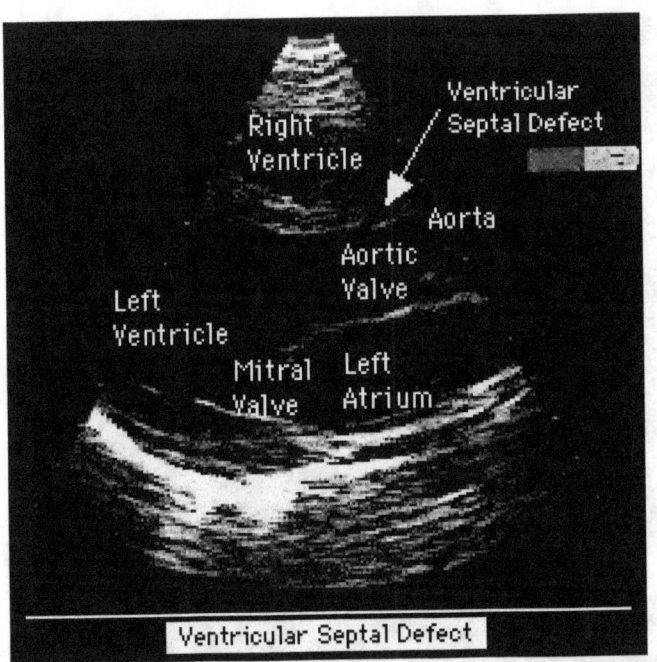

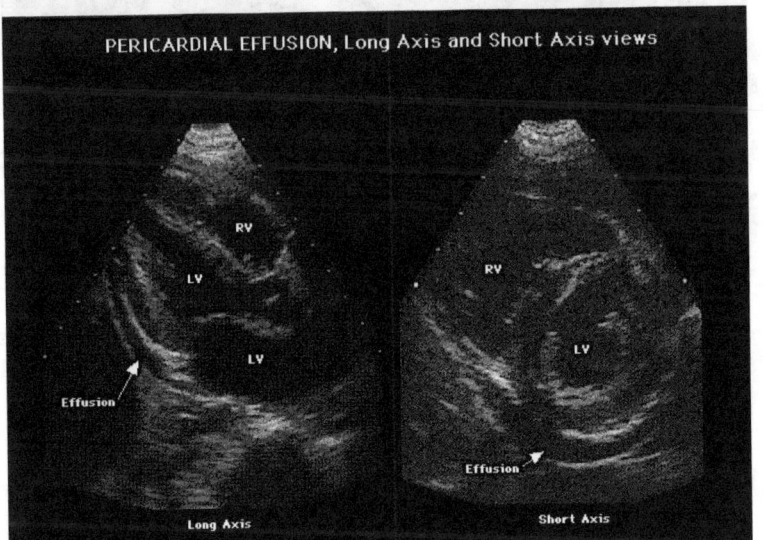

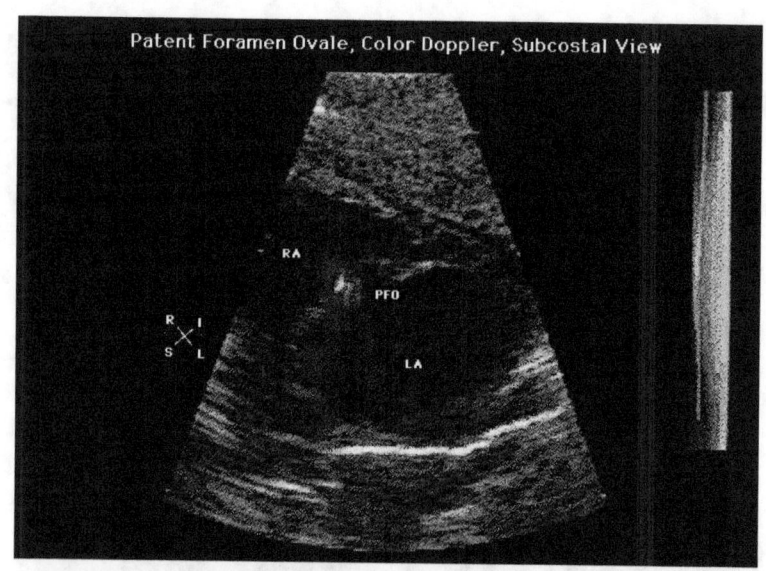

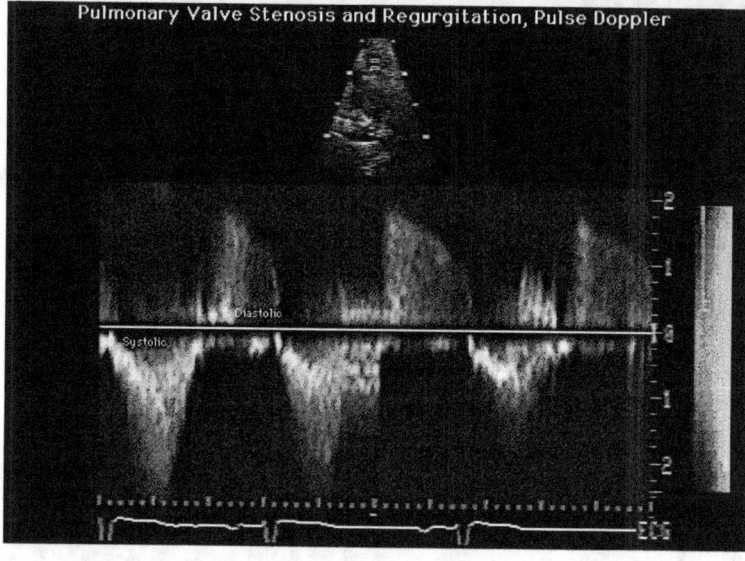

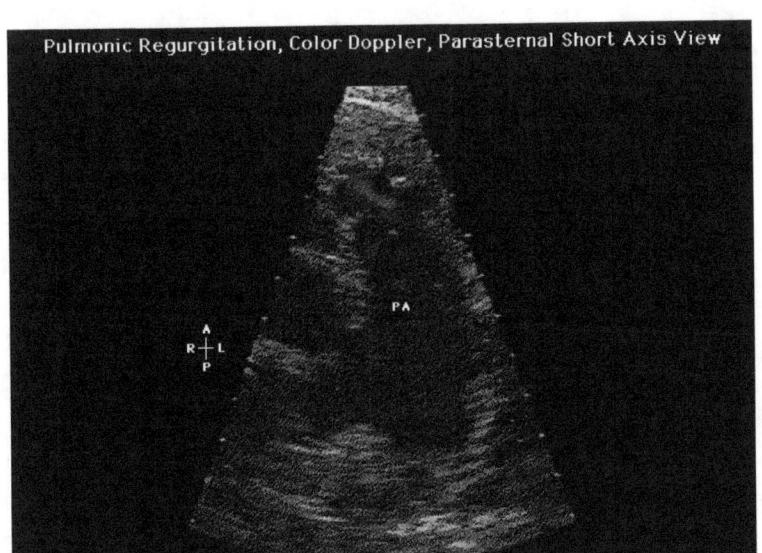

Pulmonic Regurgitation, Color Doppler, Parasternal Short Axis View

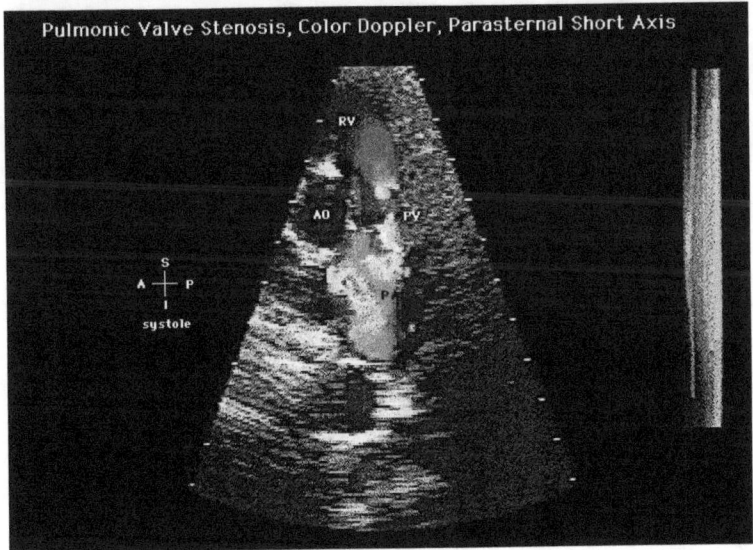

Pulmonic Valve Stenosis, Color Doppler, Parasternal Short Axis

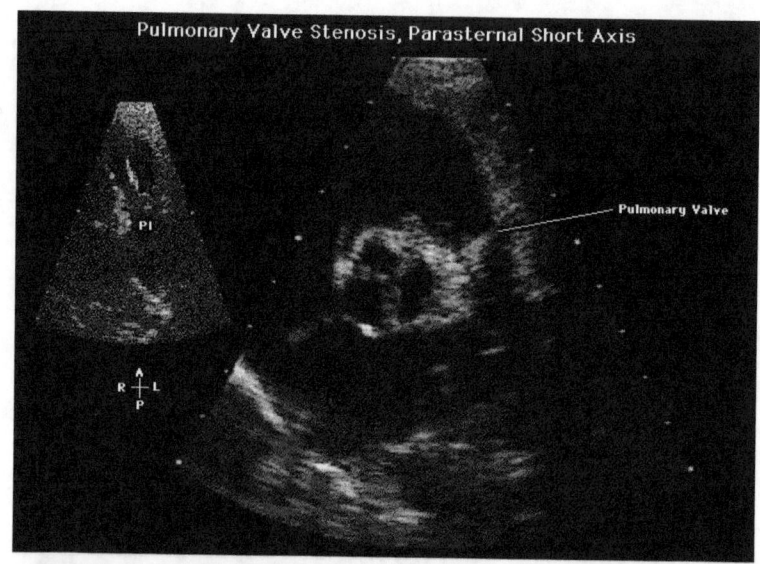
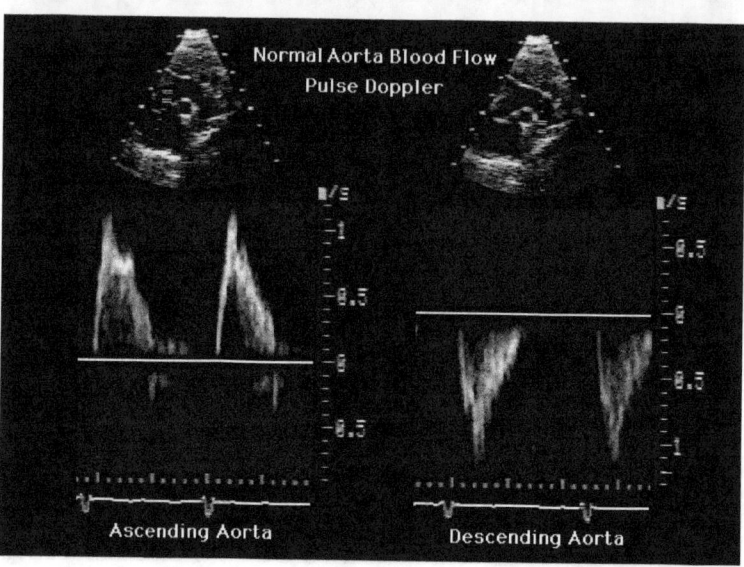

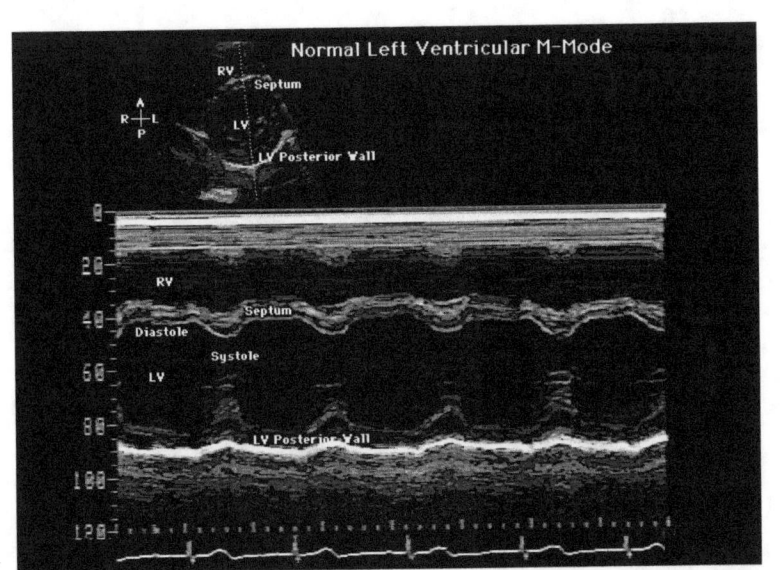

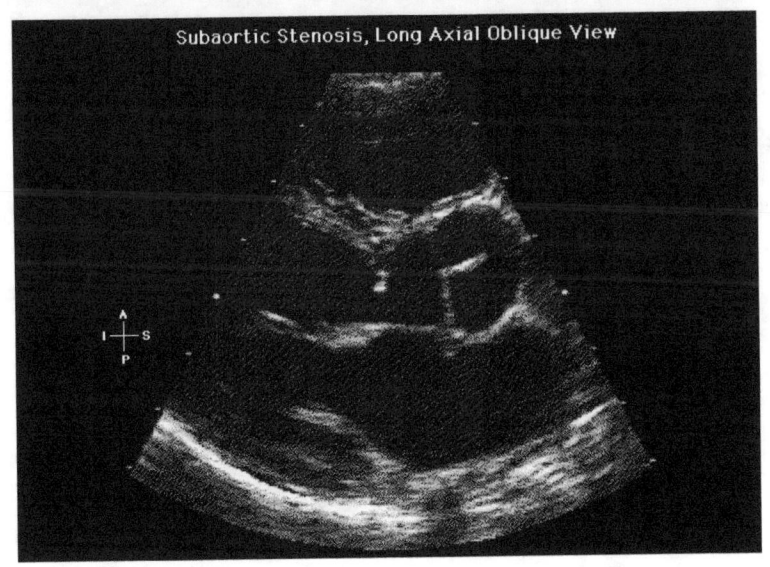

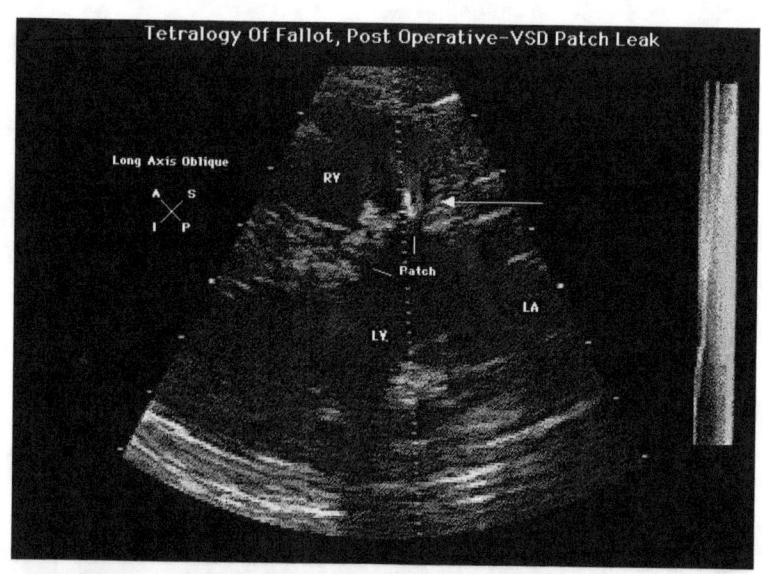

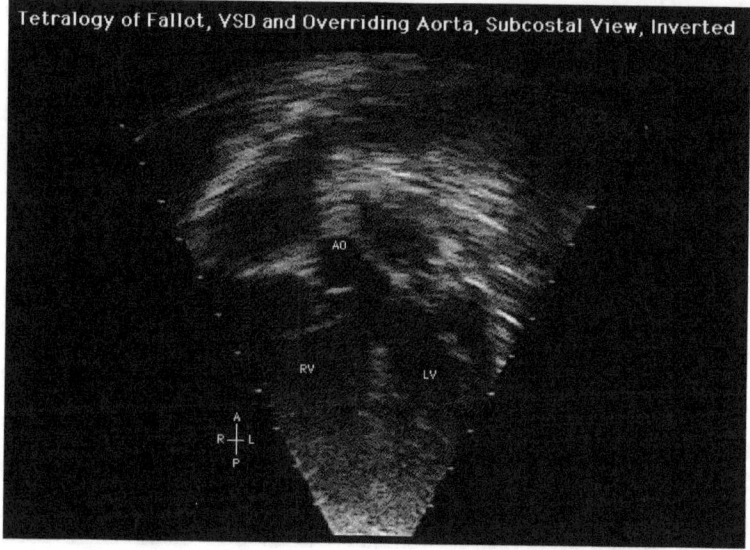

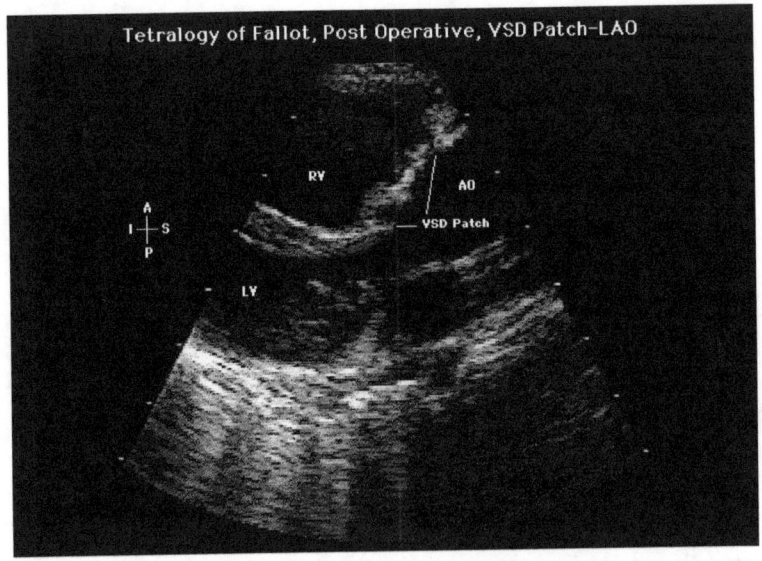

The use of Echocardiography is constantly undergoing changes and improvement. When I was in medical school I listened to my professors talk about using B-mode when it was first developed and we learned how to interpret those images.

By the time I entered my Cardiology Fellowship in 1989 color flow imaging was being introduced and we made M-mode measurements using our ECG calipers from long strips of papers recorded by the echocardiographers. By the time I finished my Fellowship in 1992 we were doing Trans Esophageal Echo (TEE) and we were beginning to use contrast bubble agents to look for atrial septal defects (ASDs) and other anomalies.

Multiple improvements have occurred since and there is no reason to believe further improvements are not on the way. Along with other imaging modalities echocardiography provides the clinician with an extremely useful tool for diagnosis and disease management.

It is my hope that this book provides you some insights into clinical echocardiography and what you can expect to see as you take care of Cardiac patients.

www.ingramcontent.com/pod-product-compliance
Lightning Source LLC
Chambersburg PA
CBHW070846220526
45466CB00002B/898